How To Seduce Hot Girls

HTeBooks

Disclaimer

This book is designed to provide condensed information. It is not intended to reprint all the information that is otherwise available, but instead to complement, amplify and supplement other texts. You are urged to read all the available material, learn as much as possible and tailor the information to your individual needs.

Every effort has been made to make this book as complete and as accurate as possible. However, there may be mistakes, both typographical and in content. Therefore, this text should be used only as a general guide and not as the ultimate source of information. The purpose of this book is to educate.

The author or the publisher shall have neither liability nor responsibility to any person or entity regarding any loss or damage caused, or alleged to have been caused, directly or indirectly, by the information contained in this book.

Table of Contents

How Will This Book Help You?

It's hard enough getting to know any random girl you cross paths with. However you don't want to just talk to the girl. You want to seduce her. You want her to fall head over heels. You want her to obediently do any number of things you ask her too, kinky or otherwise, with a smile. And you don't want just any girl. You want the hottest chicks in the bar; the most sought after coworker; your hard assed female boss who puts Kim Kardashian's assets to shame; that old high school crush you happened to come across with, and so on.

This book is here to teach you how it's done, and done right! The assumption is, you are a total newbie, you are a bumbling mess when you come across hot chicks i.e. sweaty palms, eyes looking sown on the floor; unintelligible words coming out of your mouth, heck, you might even stumble while walking away.

To be blunt, if you want to seduce hot chicks, then there are no half measures. If you are reading this, and thinking, I'll try some of the advice, then you'll most probably fail. The proper mindset for seduction success is confidence, perseverance, and a you only live once, attitude.

The basic requirements for seduction as set forth in this book are simple. First, you need to evaluate yourself. Second, you need to improve on your current self. Third, you need to know the best fishing holes. Fourth, be prepared to strike out and strike out a lot. Fifth, learn from your mistakes! Sixth, evolve into a top predator!

Why should you listen to me? Simple, I am an average guy; average face value, built, height, weight, income bracket, etc. The only thing that isn't average is the number of women I've seduced, led on, slept with, etc. When I first started out I had a batting average of 1 out of 10. Now, it's closer to 8 out of 10 successful seductions.

Don't expect this book to be a "How I Met your Mother" playbook kind of thing. It's good for a laugh, but in reality, the dating scene doesn't work like that. And most of those plays are time consuming or just plain expensive!

4

This book is straight to the point, realistic and effective. All you need to do is read, understand, execute, then continue to try again as if your life depended on it! Yes, that's all it takes!

Who Am I

"People often say that this or that person has not yet found himself. But the self is not something one finds, it is something one creates."

- Thomas Szasz

The quote above shows our intent! However the journey towards creating you version 2 starts with simple introspection. For this you will need to keep a journal. It's up to you whether you want a hard copy one or an electronic journal. Just make sure to keep it secure! The estimated timeframe for you to finish this exercise is 3 to 5 days.

The Story of Your Life

Take the time to write highlights of your life, for as long as you can remember. Do it in chronological order from your youngest years to the present. The goal of this exercise is threefold. The first is for you to rediscover who it is you are exactly. The second is for you to identify key experiences that helped shape you. The third is, you can use some of these information to shape your seduction spiel later on.

Your Strengths

Look at yourself from the perspective of a third person. What are your strengths? What are you good at? There is no need to be shy and you shouldn't exaggerate your strengths either. Be very blunt and honest! Highlight strengths that you can still improve on how.

Your Weaknesses

Now for your list of weaknesses. This is going to hurt, but you need to list down everything you consider as weaknesses. Don't hold anything back. Write down ways to overcome your weaknesses. Nothing fancy or sci-fi mind you; just an honest to goodness method of self improvement list.

Hobbies and Interests

What are the things that you enjoy doing? Start with actual hobbies and interests that you are currently into. Now add other interests that you want to try out. As much as possible, start with the most realistic interests and hobbies you can literally start now. Move on to those things you want to experience in the near future, midterm, long term, etc.

Your Weekly Routine

List down in bullet form the things you actually do in a single week, what time and for how long. Do this chronologically starting from the moment you wake up to the moment you go to sleep. The goal of this exercise is to show you how much time you are actually dedicating to self improvement and how much time you are wasting away with mundane useless things like watching TV, playing video games, browsing the internet with no goal in sight, watching porn, etc.

Be detailed and honest. You are not fooling anyone here. If you do this right then self improvement becomes more manageable. Do this wrong and you end up wasting your time with half measures!

I Am Version 2.0

"You cannot dream yourself into a character; you must hammer and forge yourself one."

- James A. Froude

Now it's time to get to work! Before you even go out and talk to women, you need to be the best version of yourself. This means a transformation of sorts. The estimated timeframe for you to beta test this new version of yourself is 1 to 2 weeks. Why beta test? Well, to speed up the process you want to improve yourself a little bit then get some firsthand experience. By doing so, you let experience dictate your next move.

Physical Appearance

The best you can do in 1 to 2 weeks is to clean yourself up: get a proper haircut; shower, shave or trim your facial hair; scrub your skin clean, cut your nails; exfoliate; fix/whiten your teeth, etc. You know what, just simplify the whole experience and just go to a spa and pamper yourself with some massage, face and body scrub and a massage.

Hair

Should you change hairstyles and facial hair style? The simple answer is yes. Just don't do anything drastic. In any case hair grows back. Tip: go to a different barber and ask for a haircut. Something new, that looks good on you, and easy to maintain. Ask the barber's opinion on your facial hair, or the lack of it.

Skin

If you are too white for your own good, go out and get a tan. If you are backed by the sun, exfoliate to get rid of dull dead skin cells.

Smell

Women have a finely developed sense of smell. The easiest way to turn off a woman is to stink. Cover all your smell bases. This includes your breath; hair; perfume; armpits, feet, crotch area. Always carry mints, but if you are in a restaurant, lemon water or cinnamon infused coffee is a good breath freshener. Always shower before the deed. Don't forget to scrub your sensitive bits; gently of course.

Tip: coordinate the way you smell. Buy one of those complete Eau de cologne packages from a respectably fashionable brand i.e. Georgio Armani, Clinique, CK, Ralph Lauren, etc. You don't need to break the bank. However you do need to smell like you are a virile alpha. This is a sound investment for a man on the prowl. Remember, cold temperatures require warm musky scents while warmer temperatures require fresh citrusy scents.

Clothes

A man on the prowl needs to be well dressed. This does not mean the most expensive brands. It doesn't even mean brand new clothes. What it does mean, are clothes that fit you properly, clean, and appropriate for the occasion.

The problem with men and clothes is that you either have a sense of style or you don't. If you belong to the former, well and good. Chances are this means you've been complemented on how you wear your clothes several times already.

If you don't have a strong sense of style, then you need help. Ask friends whom you know have impeccable style. Ask for the opinion of the salesclerk. Common sense also dictates you keep things simple. Not too loose, not too tight a fit. Tip: wear something that helps you stand out in a good way. Don't overdo things mind you!

Exercise

If you want to seduce females, you want to be in good shape. This also helps with you sexual prowess and stamina. You don't need to look like one of those hunk models in the centerfold. All you need to do is to be in good shape. Of course, it would be best if you regularly keep an exercise routine, so much so that after several months, you are in the best shape of your life!

Posture

Women love men who look and feel confident. In large part, this means proper posture. This starts as a conscious effort to stand up straight; take confident strides and look at where you're going, occasionally staring momentarily and smiling at women you come across with. Work on this until it becomes a subconscious effort.

Eye Contact

Seduction is all about contact. And the first thing that makes contact is the eyes. Don't look down. Don't look to the side. Don't stare either. Look at her for a few seconds. Smile. Resist the urge to give her a head to toe glance.

Confidence is the key in seducing women. So stay calm. Take purposeful actions. Make eye contact and smile.

The Art of the Spoken Word

"Pick up Line Jokes are exactly that...jokes"

- Author Unknown

In my opinion, pick up lines that are funny, can only work for you if the girl you are seducing is already into you; or as an ice breaker. In other words, you can't expect to mumble a few choice words and expect her to want you inside of her! It takes a little bit more work than that.

If you really want to pick up women, then you need to talk. Don't talk to them like they're idiots! Don't put them in a pedestal as well. Remember, even the most gorgeous woman has to shit and wipe her ass at least once a day! They're human's too...yummy, yummy, humans, but humans nonetheless.

My Name is...

This is always the best way to start a conversation. Walk up to her, make eye contact, and introduce yourself. If upon eye contact, she smiles and is receptive to your introduction, offer your hand and shake hers. Do it in a masculine but gentle way. The important thing is to establish skin contact.

I'm New Here...

The lost puppy is a simple but effective means to get her to pay attention. This is based on science really, women have a maternal instinct to guide lost boys, and it's that simple. All you have to do is add an appropriate phrase:

"Do you know a good place to have lunch?" After she points you to a spot, you ask her, if she's tried it out herself. Whatever her answer, invite her for lunch. Make an excuse like "I hate eating alone, and

I've still got a couple of questions to ask. My treat, it's the least I could do!"

Can I buy you a drink? All it'll cost you is a few minutes of your time. This is applicable both in bars and coffee shops. Why does it work? Ask any woman out there; at one time or another they have fantasized about sitting alone in a coffee shop or a bar, and someone sweeps them off their feet. The trick is to make an impression. And you do that by being the best version of you, and being confident.

Can you point me to the right section? You can use this if you are in the library. Yes, people still go to libraries. You can also use this on the street. Don't be fresh though. Some women are just plain helpful. Say thank you and just as you are about to walk away, turn back, like an afterthought. Ask her out for coffee or lunch. If she hesitates but is clearly interested, you close the deal by saying "It's not every day you meet a stranger and have the chance to become friends. It's just coffee/lunch?"

Keep things simple and straight to the point.Making a joke is always good for a laugh. But it is always the honest answers that get you the girl!

Make a Connection

"Every good conversation starts with good listening and observation"

- Author Unknown

Let's assume she does give you a few minutes of her time. Going by experience, you have 5 minutes tops to get her interested in you. After that she will be obviously inattentive in the hopes that you give up. If she's feeling spiteful, she'll probably cut you off and ask to leave. So what can you do in five minutes? Below are a few suggestions:

Unless your day job is interesting as hell, then you do not initiate conversation about the same. If she asks, answer with a short 30 seconds to 1 minute statement.

Look at what she is wearing. Is she holding a book, a phone, her jewelry, her shoes, etc., to get an idea of what type of activity she enjoys. Don't assume and tell her, "Do you do yoga?" Insert yourself by suggesting a connection and then making her think it was her idea. For example, after this I got to get my a yoga mat. Know of any fitness hubs around here?

Don't try too hard. You want to sound interested but not desperate. For example: "I really feel a connection", sounds lame. "How about we do this some other time, maybe this coming Friday?" If she is interested she will find the time.

Say goodbye. It is important that you are the one who cuts the encounter short. Tell her, you are in a rush or that you feel guilty taking up too much of her time. By doing so, you are in the position of power. The best time to cut the conversation short is just when things get interesting. This takes a maximum of 30 minutes. Anything more and you are pushing it.

Contact info. Do you ask for her contact info or do you give her yours? Keep the ball in your court by asking her for her digits. If she seems hesitant, don't push it. How, about I give you my number instead. That way, if you do change your mind, you can always call me.

Part with a touch. Gauge the situation. If she feels cold or unsure, then part with a handshake. If she seems in too you, nodding, laughing, touching her hair, etc., you can take a risk and kiss the top of her hand very gently, then smile.

Introduce yourself, get her to agree to something you suggest, make a connection, then abruptly cut the encounter. Let her simmer for 2 days, then contact her.

Always Be Closing

Here's the situation. You get a girl interested in you. You go on a first date and its fun. You go on a second date and it's also fun. You go on a third date, but dufus that you are, you are still afraid to peck her on the cheek as a greeting. You are still afraid to take her by the shoulder and waist to share an umbrella. As a result, that initial interest in you becomes blah. She gets a second wind and realizes you are boring and not worth the time, or she starts thinking you are uninterested.

I Really Like You

"And I don't mean, I like you as a friend. To put it simply, I am attracted to you. The way you smile, your smell, your ideas..." Drive the point home by gently touching her hand. If she doesn't pull away, then you've got her.

Don't Be too Pushy

Get to know her as a person first before asking her about her personal details. This means you ask her about what she thinks about current events, where are her favorite vacation spots, where does she like to hang out, etc. Avoid taboo subjects like past relationships, how much she makes, is that a boob job, and the like.

Getting Touchy

When is the right time to stop being a relief player and start playing ball i.e. first base, second base, third base, home run, etc. Well, the answer depends on the situation and the girl. In the first case, you can control the situation by getting her in the mood: dinner, plenty of laughs, and, yes a little bit of alcohol. In the second case, well, it's a trial and error thing. The rule of thumb is, you can push your luck but don't do it in such a way that she will be offended.

Tip: it's not always easy getting some alone time with a girl. Taking her home, and asking for a tour of her apartment is usually a Hail Mary. What you can do is get the touching over with, so you can move on to more intimate acts.

Dancing Is a Necessary Skill!!!

The best way to touch her, even with plenty of people looking, is to dance with her. Personally, the author prefers slow and ballroom dancing moves. This allows you to hold her hands, touch her waist, breath on her neck, even be a few inches away from her face, looking like a maniac! There is also the simple reality that, even on the most modern clubs, ballroom dancing is a welcome act. This skill takes time to practice. Don't worry, every bit of effort you put into it is worth it!

At the end of your dance, she will be out of breath, you are smiling, and she has just gotten used to you touching her all over. Now asking to enter her apartment for some refreshments becomes easier.

Don't beat around the bush. Close the deal at the appropriate time.

Cover All Your Bases

"Practice makes perfect applies to the most mundane of things."

- Author Unknown

First Base (French Kiss)

You don't ask to kiss her. But you do give her enough leeway to mirror your move or run for the hills. The worst time to go for a kiss is immediately after an awkward moment of silence. The best time is after laughing and smiling. For example, while walking her home, make small talk and while both of you are laughing, make serious eye contact.

This is where it gets tricky. Slowly move in to kiss the girl. Stop 1 inch or so, away from her face and gauge her reaction. If she freezes but doesn't pull away; go in for the kiss. Your kiss should be full on the lips with mouth open. Now your initial motion will push her slightly backwards. Let her correct herself and push you a little bit back as well. You do this by relaxing your neck muscles. That push and pull motion will create the necessary inertia for a longer lasting kiss. It will also show her that she does in fact want you.

Second Base (Them Boobies)

Second base means you actually fondle her breasts with your bare hands. If you fondle her breast with clothing getting in between that doesn't count. Naturally the venue for such actions is limited. In most cases you do it in the car, or inside your/her apartment. On some kinky occasions, you can let the heat of the moment dictate itself and do it in a dark alley.

Considering experience, your first foray on second base will be met with resistance. That is why it is a good idea to get it over with now, so your next time will met with the green light. It's simple, if you've been locking lips for more than 5 minutes now, then it's time to put your arms around her shoulders, caress the same and slowly move lower. You then unhook her bra with a simple motion of one hand pulling down and the other pulling up.

Tip: it's not easy to unhook a bra. The problem with failing to unhook it in the very first instance means you give her time to resist your advances. How do you become proficient at unhooking a bra? Simple, you buy one and practice it at home. The mechanism and motion is the same if the bra hook is located in the back or on the side.

What if she is wearing a bra with a hook in front? How about a sports bra? In case you feel her back and side and don't find that telltale hook, then your next option is to insert one hand on the underside of her bra, directly below the a breast. Do this gently and with a cupping motion until your arms slides onto her bare breasts and the bra move up.

Third Base (Eating her Snatch)

Third base is an optional thing. Some men like to do it; other men don't want any part in it. There is also the fact that some women resist the act itself. This isn't a smut eBook so we won't go into the details for this one. Needless to say, if you are able to get her naked from the waist down, you're good enough on your own!

Home Run (Le Sexy Time)

This is the actual intimate act of sexual intercourse. Just a few pointers here: don't try to bite off more than you can chew. If you know you've got a limp biscuit, then use some Viagra, but follow the instructions. If you are no expert on sexual positions, then stick with the triumvirate of missionary, cowgirl and doggie.

Also, a woman is not an oil well, so don't pump like there's no tomorrow! Kiss her, fondle her breasts, caress her body, take it slow. By doing so, you increase your chances of a repeat performance.

Know your way around a woman's body. And, learn the basics of making love to a woman.

Hotspots

"Location, Location, Location"

- Author Unknown

Think of it this way, no matter how good you are at fishing, if you go to a dried up river bed, you won't catch anything! Finding places were females are hot and receptive to male advances isn't rocket science. But it does require you to do some leg work.

Birds of the Same Feather

It's simple; if you want to fish for college chicks, you go to a pub near a coed university. If you want to hunt for cougars you go to hotel lounges, and ballroom dancing joints. If you want yuppies, then go to a stylish bar or café. If you want the sweet and innocent kind, the local Starbucks might yield you some of that.

Camouflage

It is important that you wear clothes appropriate to the locale. Going to a pub dressed the nines with Armani might get you some stares, but you are being too obvious.

Time and Tide

Friday nights is a feeding frenzy. So if you are not yet a top predator, you better stick to weekday nights or even afternoons. You can then progress to happy hour and then Saturday nights. Remember, you are both a predator and prey. No matter how hot you are, if there is someone hotter than you, she might just decide to take a chance and see if she can bait that other more attractive male specimen.

Moving On

There are nights when you have it, there are nights when you don't. Know when to cut your losses. If this day was a bust, don't fret, there is always tomorrow. Also, if you've been chatting up a woman and she hasn't been volunteering information herself, then maybe it's time to move on. Don't push your luck too much, you might just irritate her and get noticed by other potential prey. Tip: if you crashed and burned 3 times in a single bar or joint, either call it a night or move on to another location.

Location and timing is important. Knowing when to cut your losses is also important. Remember, you didn't waste your time. You credit every unsuccessful bid to experience!

If You've Got It Flaunt It!

"Confidence is silent. Insecurities are loud"

- Author Unknown

Everybody has something they can use to pick up chicks. It can be from the very obvious like a bad ass car, awesome crib, famous friends, etc. It can also be less obvious like your pearly whites, deep dimples, your awesome singing voice or your great dance moves. The trick is to flaunt it without being too obvious. Remember, desperate does not get you laid. Below are a few things to remember.

Your Car

Be realistic here, is your car a chick magnet or a mom mobile? The worst you can do is try to dress up a minivan like a sports car. You're just trying too hard. Best keep it stock and use whatever else is under your disposal.

If you do have a chick magnet for a car, then don't treat it like it's more important than the girl you are trying to impress. Show your car but don't demand that she takes off her shoes before entering!

Your Body

The good thing about the human body is, you can pretty much change from an obese guy to a muscle bound hunk. All you really need is dedication and some whey protein.

The biggest turn off is a guy checking his guns in the mirror, or flexing his muscles without any reason. If you've got a stellar physique, then fitted shirts and leave it at that.

Also, avoid over emphasizing on one part of your body and forgetting other less desirable bits. For example, you've got ripped biceps but a pot belly!

Your Looks

If you've got a handsome mug, then you have the advantage. But for crying out loud, make absolutely sure you so have a handsome mug! The last thing you want is to have an average face value and build yourself up so much that when you do meet your blind date, she is disappointed!

The best form of bragging is subtle and sly. All you really need is to show the goods, and let it do the talking.

Get a Hobby

"Birds of the same feather, flock together"

- Cecil Thounaojam

A hobby allows you to break the monotony of day to day life. This is a very good conversation starting point. It is also a good place to meet women who have the same interest. And nowadays, even the geekiest hobby attracts hot chicks! As an added bonus, both of you already have something in common. That is one less thing to worry about.

Something You Genuinely Like!

Just to be clear, you are selecting a hobby based on what you really enjoy doing. You don't select a hobby based on how many chicks you think are interested. That defeats the purpose of the entire exercise!

You Aren't Limited to Just 1

You can have as many hobbies as you like. Although, realistically your limit will depend on your budget and the actual amount of time you can dedicate to the same.

Don't Break the Bank

You don't need to buy expensive gear, at least not at the get go. Start with the basics. Buy smaller stuff. Save up for big ticket purchases.

A hobby makes you more interesting. It also allows you to meet people you actually share an interest with.

Last Minute Tips

"Simplicity and Truth is Key to Happiness"

- Author Unknown

Dating and picking up chicks is for your pleasure and happiness. That is a simple fact that you should always remember. Some guys tend to get too caught up in the game that they forget this. So much so that they lie, cheat, make up complications that could have easily been avoided. Below are a few points to remember.

Exaggerate But Don't Lie

Let's be honest, when picking up chicks you tend to exaggerate, or at the very least put the best foot forward. There is nothing wrong with that, provided you keep things reasonable. The problem starts when you rely on outright lies to get her attention. For one thing, lying is complex and hard work. If you lie about one thing, there is a tendency to continue lying just to cover up your earlier fib.

Internet Dating

Use the internet to your advantage. There is no harm in trying free internet dating sites or forum based dating sites. Heck, you can literally use the same as practice for when you actually talk up to a real live woman. Just remember, that talking is free online. If a website requires you to pay membership fees or whatever they might call, it move on to another site.

Don't do Anything Stupid!

This is the internet day and age. The last thing you want is earn the ire of a woman and get your face plastered all over social media pages. Remember, you want to bang her, but it doesn't mean you should disrespect her.

When in Doubt Err on the Side of Caution

If something smells fishy, or if an offer sounds too good to be true, then perform your due diligence. Man is blessed with intuition to fight or flee. If every fiber of your being says something is wrong, then go with your gut. For example: a telltale Adams apple; scam alert; no videos please, and the like!

Don't over complicate this. You want to seduce women, not lie to them. You want to enjoy the experience not drown in a convoluted lie. And above all, keep safe and follow your gut feeling!

How to Apply What You've Learned?

Assess yourself honestly. Know your weaknesses and your strengths. Now build self confidence internally by calming your emotions and externally by purposeful action. Build rapport thru humor and sincerity.

Remember, location is always important. You need to be properly situated to get the best possible bite. Know when to cut your losses. Everyone has a bad day. Learn from your failures. These lessons are just as valuable as your successes. If you are running low on ideas or hotspots, go back to what you enjoy doing. Take up a hobby.

Now make a connection by way of your words, sense of touch, smell, and the like. When you have her on the ropes, pounce and seal the deal! Let's go someplace more private or how about a nightcap?

You've worked so hard to get her in private. Don't mess things up with fumbling fingers, and a wham bam thank you ma'am attitude. Make love to her. Enjoy her body to the fullest!